AF483357

ABOUT THIS WORKBOOK

This workbook is designed to dive deeper into each of the Seven Sacred Truths.

We came into human form to learn and experience the richness of a full life. As part of this full life, we have inherited dysfunctional belief systems from generations before us, which can sometimes cause us to live in the shadow of our truest selves.

Through Help in Healing suggestions & Journal Questions, you will be guided to unpack & explore what is drawing you out of alignment and out of your truth.

I encourage you to explore each question with love, compassion, and nurturing for your sweet self.

Reflect on the questions with complete honesty and, equally important—*without* self-judgment or shame.

My goal in writing this book was to raise the vibration of this extraordinary planet one beautiful person at a time.

I want you to live your very best life. And to do that, you must *Stand in Your Truth!*

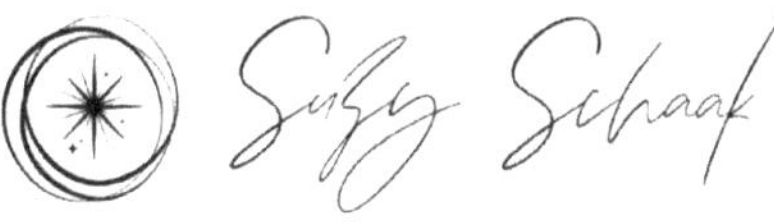

STAND IN YOUR TRUTH: SEVEN SACRED TRUTHS TO LIVING A DIVINELY GUIDED LIFE

ISBN: 979-8-218-41751-2

DIVINE MANIFESTATION

Let's get grounded in your beautiful body and explore your foundational beliefs.

DIVINE REBIRTH

Step into your power, and let's create!

DIVINE WILL

By surrendering, we allow the will of Divinity to guide our path.

DIVINE LOVE

Bridge the love within your physical experience with that of the Divine.

DIVINE TRANSFORMATION

Discover how every breath you take and every thought you create transforms your life experience.

DIVINE WISDOM

Allow your body's wisdom to awaken the wisdom of the Divine, understanding that we are one living consciousness.

DIVINE LIGHT

Remember who you are!

LET'S MANIFEST

Create the life of your dreams!

Divine Manifestation

"When your vibration becomes love, those around you share in this love vibration so that everything around you moves into a place of constant sacred manifestation." –BT

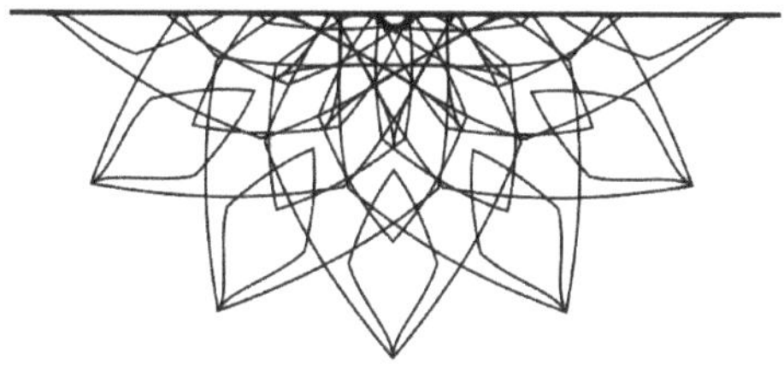

"I am the Light of Divine Manifestation. Through this Sacred Truth, I have a knowingness that I am safe and deeply grounded to Mother Earth. I am a sacred vessel, cradling and nurturing my Soul Light of Divinity within me."

Help in Healing

The intention of Divine Manifestation is to create an energetic vessel to hold and ground Divine Light and Love in the sacredness of your physical body.

BE STILL & LISTEN!

Carve out time each day to just be alone with yourself and Spirit. Tune into the wisdom that comes forward. Everyone receives this insight differently, so be patient with yourself and see how your inner voice shares its story. What is your body's wisdom expressing?

SHIFT YOUR PERSPECTIVE

As you observe your experiences, be a witness rather than a participant to discern these experiences in your life objectively. What do you notice when you are the observer rather than being attached to the situation or the outcome?

CONNECT TO THE EARTH

When I feel out of sorts or chaotic, I have learned that the best way for me to find my center is to take a forest walk, and to stand barefoot in the grass, or, even better, mud. This allows me to feel the vibration of the earth. What helps you to best connect?

GIVE AND RECEIVE THE GIFT OF TOUCH

One of my favorite ways to get grounded and feel supported is through a long hug or holding hands with a loved one. That is the gift we enjoy by living in a human body. How do you feel when you have physical touch with another beautiful being, whether it be on the giving or receiving end or both?

NATURE PROVIDES US WITH UNCONDITIONAL LOVE

Find some stillness on your walk and take in the earth's vibration. Surrender what isn't serving you and just receive. How does your body respond to beautiful Mother Earth?

TRY GARDENING AND EAT GROUNDING FOODS

There's an amazing difference when we actually grow our own food and get our hands in the dirt. We've poured love into the plants, and they offer that love and nutrition in return. What types of food nurture and ground you?

TAKE TIME FOR A GROUNDING BREATH & MEDITATION

Be present with your body and feel your connection to the earth. By incorporating these throughout the day and before bed, how do you feel this will impact your stress levels and quality of sleep?

WHAT ELSE CONNECTS YOU TO YOUR BODY?

It is so important to stay connected to our bodies and listen to their wisdom. Cues from your body are your best way to keep it healthy and happy. Remember...listen when it's a whisper rather than a roar.

ADDITIONAL THOUGHTS & FEELINGS

ADDITIONAL THOUGHTS & FEELINGS

ADDITIONAL THOUGHTS & FEELINGS

Journal Questions

Let's take a deeper dive. As you ponder each question, ask yourself, "Am I being honest with myself?" This can be a lovely conversation between yourself and Spirit. Spirit knows all the answers and is compassionate and patient as you find the courage to face the truth in your answers.

DOES YOUR FOUNDATION HAVE ANY CRACKS (PAST OR PRESENT) THAT NEED YOUR ATTENTION?

Think of your foundational needs, such as safety, security, & love.

ARE YOU MEETING YOUR FOUNDATIONAL NEEDS?

If not, what are actionable steps you can take to make this happen?

DO YOU FEEL GROUNDED, STABLE, & SAFE?

Can you define the areas in your life that feel or felt unstable and the time in which they occurred? This is helpful in beginning your healing journey, as it allows you to understand how deeply rooted they are and how much they have impacted the rest of your life.

DO YOU FEEL LOVED BY YOURSELF & OTHERS? IF NOT, WHY NOT?

You are deserving of love. When I see a client in the healing room, I have the privilege of witnessing their Soul's perfection. No matter what has happened to you in your life or what you have done, you are perfect, and the essence of who you are is love.

DO YOU ACCEPT LOVE FROM YOURSELF AND OTHERS? IF NOT, WHY NOT?

If your answer is no, reflect back on when and why this began. Scope out and observe yourself as a small child. What would you tell this beautiful child that is you?

IS THERE WOUNDING THAT REQUIRES YOUR LOVE AND ATTENTION?

Take some time to name and describe the wounding. Once you truly know what it is, you can begin to address it.

DO YOU NEED HELP EXPLORING THIS WOUNDING? IF SO, WHO CAN YOU REACH OUT TO?

First, call in your angels and Spirit Guides. They are just waiting to step in and support you. Also, consider reaching out for support from a trusted friend, family member, support group, mental health care provider, or me. Please know that you are never alone. If shame or fear is getting in your way, name it, and remember you are absolute perfection and deserve to feel joy and love.

ADDITIONAL THOUGHTS & FEELINGS

ADDITIONAL THOUGHTS & FEELINGS

ADDITIONAL THOUGHTS & FEELINGS

ADDITIONAL THOUGHTS & FEELINGS

ADDITIONAL THOUGHTS & FEELINGS

Divine Rebirth

"Divine Rebirth means that every day, out of love for yourself, out of love for the sacredness of who you are, you must tend to the Divinity and that of the blessed life force that is continually generating within you." –BT

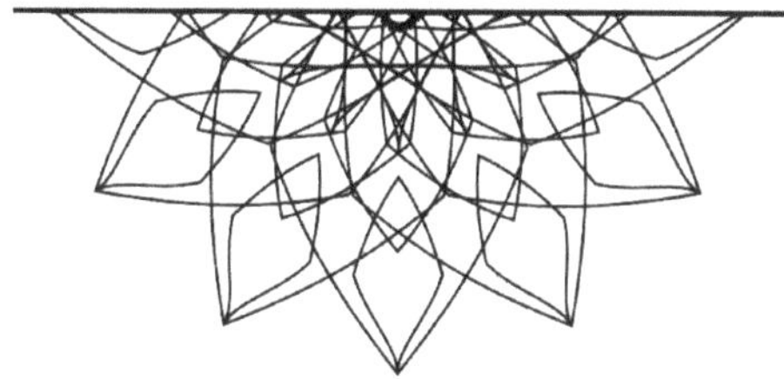

"I am the Light of Divine Rebirth. Through this Sacred Truth, I have the potential to transform, regenerate, renew, and reawaken all things."

Help in Healing

Divine Rebirth is about evolving and shape-shifting in and out of our comfort zone. Whether it's personal transformation and enlightenment within, discovering your life's purpose, manifesting better health, a new relationship, career, or home, let's explore Divine Rebirth, plant the seeds of change, and give birth to something new.

SIMPLIFY YOUR LIFE

Take a look at your life and see where your time, energy, and resources are being spent.

- What do you love? What are non-negotiables in terms of relationships, activities, and financial commitments?
- What friendships/relationships and commitments are no longer serving you?
- What financial burdens can you release?
- Is there anything else that is taking up unnecessary space in your life?

Remember to pause and deeply reflect on these answers because they will liberate you from your current situation.

ADDITIONAL THOUGHTS & FEELINGS

RECOGNIZE & RELEASE EMOTIONAL ATTACHMENTS

What attachments do you have to things, people, and titles? Attachments are usually rooted in ego or fear, and that is what keeps us attached. Often, we don't feel safe, good enough, or strong enough to release them. Take time to be really honest with yourself when answering this.

FREE YOURSELF FROM FINANCIAL BURDENS—A DEEPER DIVE

Are there ways you can simplify your finances (i.e., downsizing your current living situation, buying a cheaper car, recognizing your shopping habits) Are you a stress or gratification shopper?

MAKE A LIST OF WANTS VS NEEDS

This can be an eye-opener when you really take the time to dig in and be honest about those attachments.

CONSIDER INVESTING IN EXPERIENCES OVER MATERIAL POSSESSIONS

Make a list of some things you have always wanted to do, see, or experience. Then make a plan TO DO THEM!

REACH OUT FOR HELP CLEARING LIMITING BELIEFS

Let's begin by making a list of those beliefs that hold you back from living your best life. If you feel these beliefs are rooted so deeply that you don't know how to clear them, get some help from a professional.

A LACK OF CONTROL MAY BE HOLDING YOU BACK

When we feel like we must control a situation, that means there is some fear of the unknown outcome. What situations do you feel like you need to control, and why?

EXPLORE WHAT CHALLENGES YOU WITH DECISION MAKING

Remember–no decision is still a choice. When I am working with a client in the healing room who is struggling with a choice, I am guided to look at their fears and then remind them that no matter what choice they make, there is an opportunity for wisdom and growth to come forward. What challenges you?

FEELING ANXIOUS OFTEN GETS IN THE WAY OF CREATING CHANGE

Take some time to explore the root of your fears.

CO-DEPENDENCY MAKES IT DIFFICULT TO DO THINGS ON YOUR OWN & TRUST YOUR DECISION-MAKING

Is there a co-dependent relationship holding you back from trusting yourself?

ADDITIONAL THOUGHTS & FEELINGS

ADDITIONAL THOUGHTS & FEELINGS

ADDITIONAL THOUGHTS & FEELINGS

ADDITIONAL THOUGHTS & FEELINGS

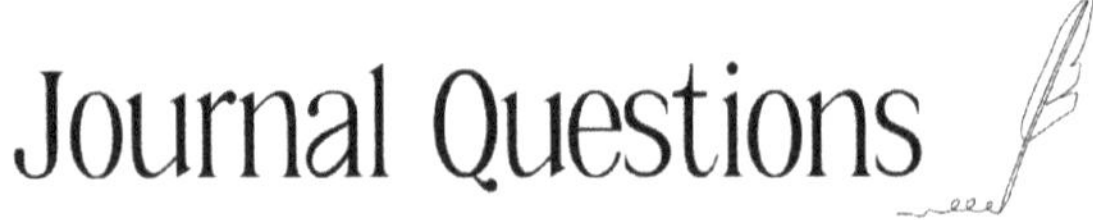

Journal Questions

DO YOU REMEMBER A TIME IN YOUR LIFE WHEN YOU FELT THE MOST POWERFUL?

There may be a few times in your life that come to mind. Journal about how this felt. Find pictures that remind you of this powerful time and put them in places where you will see them daily.

CAN YOU DESCRIBE WHAT MADE YOU THAT POWERFUL PERSON?

Remember—that powerful person is still inside of you. Take time to write about what you felt like in that experience and why you felt that way.

WHILE YOU ARE REMEMBERING YOUR POWERFUL SELF, CAN YOU BEGIN TO DAYDREAM ABOUT WHAT YOU DESIRE?

Remember—your vibration is attuned to how you feel in the present moment, whether you're remembering a past event or experiencing it in real-time. Just allow your thoughts to flow.

DOES YOUR EGO GET IN THE WAY WHILE YOU ARE DAYDREAMING?

Oftentimes, the ego will kick in with limiting beliefs, making us feel unworthy of our desires. What are your limiting beliefs?

ONCE YOU'VE DISCOVERED THE ORIGIN OF YOUR LIMITING BELIEFS, HOW CAN YOU NEUTRALIZE OR RELEASE THEM?

Remember, this is just fear coming forward, and these are simply beliefs, not your truth!

DO YOU ASK FOR ASSISTANCE FROM YOUR HIGH-VIBE TRIBE?

Your Angels, Guides, Spirit, and loved ones who have crossed are always ready to support you. But...YOU NEED TO ASK. Who is your High-Vibe Tribe? Write down what you need help in manifesting, and ask for their assistance.

ADDITIONAL THOUGHTS & FEELINGS

ADDITIONAL THOUGHTS & FEELINGS

ADDITIONAL THOUGHTS & FEELINGS

ADDITIONAL THOUGHTS & FEELINGS

Divine Will

"Divine Will is to surrender ego into the Light of Divinity and the love of the Universe." –BT

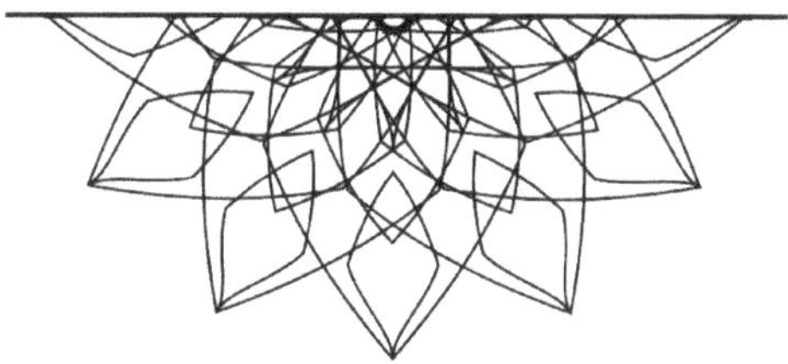

"I am the Light of Divine Will. Through this Sacred Truth, I am able to supersede my ego and surrender to the wisdom of my Divinity, allowing me to feel the beauty, bliss, and perfection in all things."

Help in Healing

Divine Will means emptying your mind of the lower ego and moving into Divine Knowingness. This beautiful Truth is about discerning when one's ego—specifically its fears, beliefs, and attachments—is superseding. When you are empowered by Divine Will, self-conflict transforms into purity and love for the world and yourself.

TAKE INVENTORY OF YOUR LIFE

What areas of your life are you trying to control?

VALIDATE YOUR FEELINGS & STRUGGLES BY GIVING EACH BURDEN A NAME

Can you begin to unload your backpack and take an honest look at what you have been carrying around?

RECOGNIZE WHAT IS YOUR RESPONSIBILITY & WHAT REQUIRES YOUR ATTENTION

What may be holding you back from taking responsibility? Can you step through the fear and acknowledge what needs your attention?

SURRENDER, SURRENDER, SURRENDER

What do you need to surrender? Are you having difficulty surrendering? Once again, call your High-Vibe Tribe for assistance with this. You may not know how to do it, so ask for help in releasing all egoic attachments.

PAUSE & BE STILL | ALLOW RATHER THAN FIGHT

Can you feel Spirit's presence in the stillness? Remember the phrase, "Not my will, but Thine be done."

- Allow all of your feelings to come forward and begin to release them.
- Journal any thoughts or feelings, or simply sit in the presence of the angels as they nurture you through this.

ADDITIONAL THOUGHTS & FEELINGS

ADDITIONAL THOUGHTS & FEELINGS

ADDITIONAL THOUGHTS & FEELINGS

Journal Questions

ARE YOU FEELING PAIN, OR HAS IT CROSSED OVER TO SUFFERING?

Remember, pain is inevitable, but suffering does not have to be.

WHAT ARE YOU ATTACHED TO IN THE SITUATION THAT IS CAUSING SUFFERING?

An attachment isn't a fact or truth. It is a belief system that can create a false and weakened sense of Self.

WHAT IS GOING ON IN YOUR LIFE THAT YOU FEEL YOU NEED TO CONTROL?

Can you pause and scope out of the situation to gain a better perspective as an observer rather than the participant?

CAN YOU SEE THE BEAUTY OR THE GIFT THROUGH THE PAIN?

Even in the most painful situations, beauty can be found. If the situation is raw, allow yourself time and space.

WHAT CHANGES ARE GOING ON IN YOUR LIFE THAT YOU MAY BE RESISTING?

Be kind and gentle with yourself as you consider this question.

HOW DO YOU FEEL ABOUT SURRENDERING WHAT YOU CANNOT CONTROL?

Take a moment to imagine what it feels like to let all the balls drop. There is something so liberating about allowing Spirit to come in and take over.

WHAT ARE YOU TRYING TO FIX?

Consider whether this needs fixing. And is fixing another way of controlling?

HOW DOES IT FEEL TO ALLOW THE SITUATION TO BE JUST AS IT IS?

Even better, can you look at the situation, whether it be a person or circumstance, as having its own Divine Plan/Wisdom?

ADDITIONAL THOUGHTS & FEELINGS

ADDITIONAL THOUGHTS & FEELINGS

ADDITIONAL THOUGHTS & FEELINGS

Divine Love

"In honoring the Light of Divinity that resides within me,
I embody The Light of Divine Love
The Light and the Love of Divine Truth
The Light and Love of Creation
The Light and Love that illumines all beings
The Light and Love of the eternal
The Light and Love that guides all souls to infinite bliss." –BT

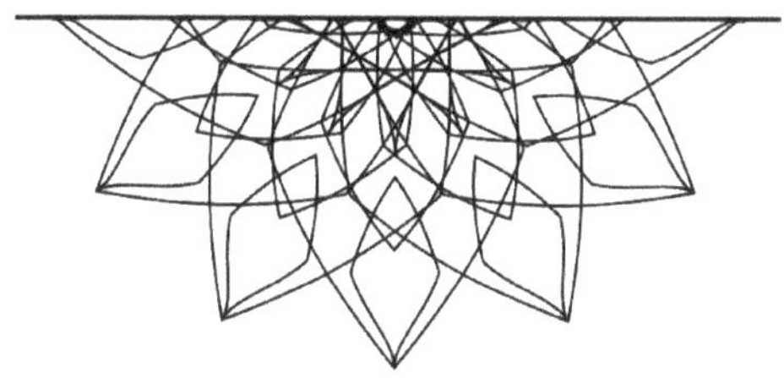

"I am Divine Love. Through this Sacred Truth, I remember that the Light within my heart supersedes all fear and heals through unconditional love."

Help in Healing

Divine Love is our moral and spiritual compass. Therefore, we must be sure all of our intentions are firmly rooted and aligned with this Sacred Truth. Holding this intention moves us beyond egoic will and into a place of humble and blessed devotion to our sacred divinity.

REMEMBER, THE DIVINE ESSENCE OF WHO YOU ARE IS LOVE.

This means that your "beingness" is love—not as an action or an emotion. You and your soul *are* love, and that is why I look at every individual as perfect.

Close your eyes and feel what I am saying. This doesn't mean that we don't step out of alignment and make mistakes. What it does mean is that stepping out of alignment doesn't diminish your perfection because you cannot strip love from your soul—they are one and the same.

Can you identify areas in your life where you are living out of alignment and have not found grace and love for yourself or others?

ADDITIONAL THOUGHTS & FEELINGS

KNOW LOVE FOR ONESELF AND OTHERS

Are you able to look into the mirror and say, "I love you!" to yourself? Do you struggle to say it to others? If so, explore what is getting in the way. Often, it's the emotion of shame. Be kind and gentle, and reflect on this last statement. Are you holding on to shame or any other lower emotions that prevent you from seeing the love and perfection that is you?

UNDERSTAND COMPASSION & EMPATHY WITHOUT PITY

Compassion and empathy feel like a warm hug. They let someone know you are feeling their pain and supporting their journey. Feeling pity for someone diminishes their experience rather than empowers them. Feel into the difference and reflect on your experiences with yourself and others.

GIVE AND RECEIVE FORGIVENESS, ACCEPTANCE, GRATITUDE, AND APPRECIATION

The truth is that forgiveness will set you free. Once you find forgiveness, only then can acceptance, gratitude, and appreciation be awakened. Is there a relationship either with yourself or someone else that deserves some forgiveness? When I struggle with this, I must scope out as the observer to see what is keeping me stuck.

PRACTICE SELF-COMPASSION AND FORGIVENESS

Above all else, these emotions need to come from within yourself. How often do you show yourself compassion and forgiveness, and how does this feel?

SPEAK TO YOURSELF WITH LOVING KINDNESS AND ALLOW YOURSELF TO FEEL ANYTHING AND EVERYTHING WITHOUT JUDGMENT

- How does your internal voice speak to you?
- Do you acknowledge and honor your feelings with respect?
- Take some time of stillness and silence to observe, and then allow your heart and Spirit to communicate its wisdom.

CULTIVATE ACCEPTANCE OF YOUR EMOTIONS—EVERY EMOTION IS SACRED AND DESERVES TO BE HEARD AND VALIDATED

Are you open to what comes from within? Do you allow yourself time and space to process everything you uncover?

ALLOW YOURSELF TIME TO GRIEVE

There is no time limit when it comes to grief. Offer yourself grace and allow the process to unfold as it needs to.

There's a delicate balance when walking through grief. We need to continue moving forward but also acknowledge that the emotion is present and allow it to be heard.

If you are walking through grief right now, are you allowing yourself time and space to feel and release and also continue to seek joy and be present in your life?

PRACTICE SELF-CARE

What are some of your self-care routines?

What allows you to let down and feel calm?

Here are some suggestions:

- Take a warm bath with rose water
- Go on a long walk
- Practice slow flow or restorative yoga
- Buy yourself some flowers or a beautiful plant
- Create a sacred space in your home for meditation and reflective time
- Try equal parts breathing (Inhale—"I am love." Exhale—gratitude)
- Speak with a trusted friend or counselor

ADDITIONAL THOUGHTS & FEELINGS

ADDITIONAL THOUGHTS & FEELINGS

ADDITIONAL THOUGHTS & FEELINGS

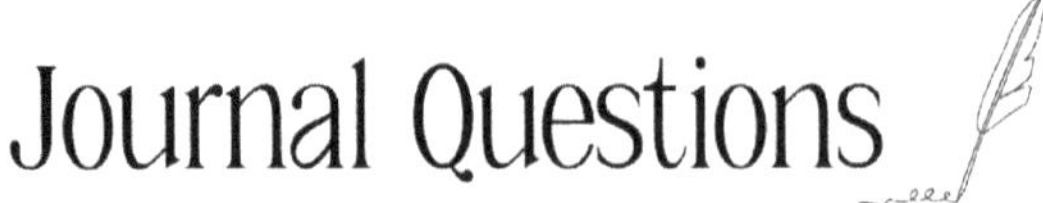

Journal Questions

WRITE YOURSELF A LOVE LETTER

Find a special card or stationary or use the space below and express all the things you appreciate and adore about yourself. Put it in a place that you will read often.

WHAT ARE SOME QUESTIONS THAT YOU HAVE HELD CLOSE TO YOUR HEART AND WOULD SERVE YOU TO EXPLORE?

Be kind and thoughtful as you begin to open your heart.

ARE THERE SOME OLD WOUNDS THAT YOU HAVE INHERITED FROM FAMILY OR DEEP RELATIONSHIPS THAT NEED EXPLORING?

Take the time and care to separate what is your responsibility in these wounds and what belongs to someone else.

ARE YOU FINDING A BALANCE BETWEEN GIVING AND RECEIVING?

- Notice your patterns. Are you giving away more than you can afford to give?
- Do you feel that you are worthy of receiving love? If not, why not?

ARE YOU TAKING MORE THAN YOU FEEL YOU SHOULD BE IN RELATIONSHIPS?

When we are taking more than giving, the emotion of guilt often shows up.

WHAT ARE SOME NURTURING WORDS OF WISDOM YOU COULD SHARE WITH YOUR BEAUTIFUL SELF?

Think of what an angel would say to you, and be that angelic light for yourself.

ADDITIONAL THOUGHTS & FEELINGS

ADDITIONAL THOUGHTS & FEELINGS

ADDITIONAL THOUGHTS & FEELINGS

ADDITIONAL THOUGHTS & FEELINGS

Divine Transformation

"Every breath you take is consciously inspired into your body as a vehicle for Divine and awakened transformation." –BT

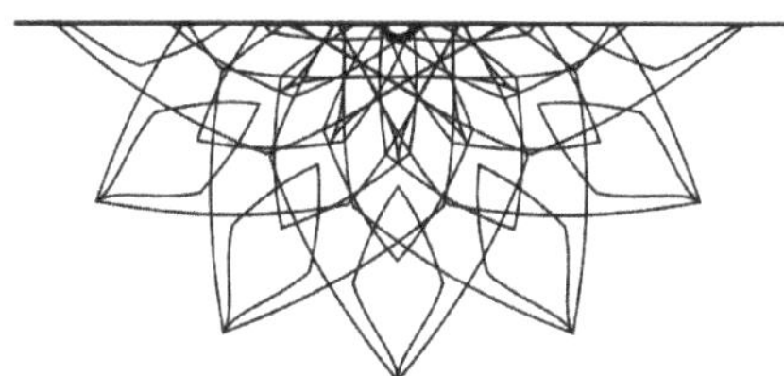

"I am the Light of Divine Transformation and self-expression. Through this truth, I know I have the ability to transform because within each breath is the Light of Spirit, and every word I speak holds the resonance of love and compassion."

Help in Healing 

Divine Transformation is a beautiful dance between Spirit and our soul, allowing your body to physically and Spiritually recreate, realign, and rejuvenate with every single breath. Think of your breath as the channel for Divine Light to move in and out of the body.

CONNECT LOVING THOUGHTS INTO YOUR WORDS

Our thoughts hold a vibration as strongly as our words. The more attention we give them, the stronger the vibration. Can you feel the difference in your physical body when your thoughts are based in love versus lower emotions?

WHEN WE'RE OUT OF ALIGNMENT, OUR THOUGHTS MANIFEST AS GOSSIP, NERVOUS CHATTER, AND AN INABILITY TO SEE EACH OTHER THROUGH A LENS OF LOVE

Close your eyes and visualize what that vibration looks like. How does that vibration impact your physical and mental health?

IMAGINE IF YOU WERE ABLE TO BECOME FLUENT IN RECOGNIZING IMMEDIATELY WHEN YOUR THOUGHTS STEPPED OUT OF ALIGNMENT

What are some steps you can take so that you become aware immediately?

IF YOU FIND YOURSELF IN A DISAGREEMENT OR SIMPLY DO NOT FEEL SEEN OR HEARD, TAKE A MOMENT TO BREATHE INTO YOUR BEAUTIFUL BODY

- Can you feel yourself filling with Divine Light?
- Can you lift yourself out of the situation and see it as an observer rather than a participant?
- How does your perspective shift?

TAKE A MOMENT TO REFLECT ON CONFLICT IN YOUR LIFE AS AN OBSERVER

- Are you able to own what is your responsibility and see more clearly what is not?
- Can you take steps to heal what you are responsible for?
- Can you release what is not by finding compassion and grace for yourself, the situation, and anyone involved?

OBSERVE HOW YOU CAN HEAL THROUGH YOUR BREATH

Visualize what Divine Light looks like as it enters your body. How would you describe it and how does it feel?

PRACTICE PRANAYAMA DAILY

- Check out my Meditations on the Suzy Schaak Yoga YouTube page.
- Try doing the Ribbon Of Light Meditation.
- What breathing exercises work the best for your body?

ADDITIONAL THOUGHTS & FEELINGS

ADDITIONAL THOUGHTS & FEELINGS

ADDITIONAL THOUGHTS & FEELINGS

ADDITIONAL THOUGHTS & FEELINGS

Journal Questions

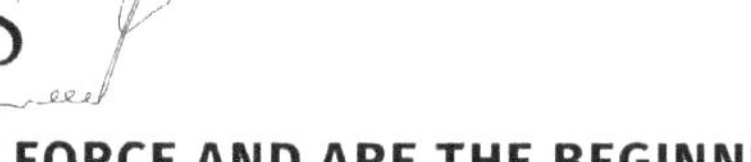

YOUR THOUGHTS TAKE ON A LIFE FORCE AND ARE THE BEGINNING STAGES OF MANIFESTATION

- How do you speak to yourself?
- What does your internal dialogue look and feel like?

FEELINGS & UNSPOKEN WORDS HAVE A POSITIVE OR NEGATIVE VIBRATION

- What are the negative loops that keep you stuck?
- Is there a loving mantra you can create for yourself when you find yourself becoming negative? My mantra is, “I am love.”

YOU ARE AN EXTRAORDINARY, ANGELIC BEING!

Journal about at least one aspect of yourself you find beautiful.

DO YOU TAKE THINGS PERSONALLY & BEGIN TO SPIRAL WHEN A CONVERSATION DOES NOT GO SMOOTHLY?

What beliefs do you attach to these exchanges?

ARE YOU SPEAKING TO YOURSELF & OTHERS THROUGH THE LENS OF LOVE?

Do you recognize when your egoic mind steps in and derails a conversation?

IF WE LACK SELF-WORTH, WE ARE AFRAID TO BE SEEN OR HEARD AND OFTEN JUST GO ALONG WITH OTHERS

Do you feel worthy of being listened to?

THIS PATTERN ALSO SHOWS UP BY KEEPING SECRETS

- What thoughts and feelings have you kept hidden?
- Can you begin to let them out by journaling about them?
- Are you afraid to be honest with yourself about your thoughts and beliefs?

AFTER DOING THE BREATHING EXERCISE I SHARED, HOW DID THIS MAKE YOUR BODY FEEL?

- As you partake in this breathing exercise, what is coming forward for you? Do you feel emotional or physical discomfort as you release through the breathing exercise?
- Can you trace it back to its origin and begin to heal it?

HOW DOES IT MAKE YOUR BODY FEEL WHEN YOU ALLOW IT TO BREATHE DEEPLY?

How does this make your Spirit feel?

ADDITIONAL THOUGHTS & FEELINGS

ADDITIONAL THOUGHTS & FEELINGS

ADDITIONAL THOUGHTS & FEELINGS

ADDITIONAL THOUGHTS & FEELINGS

Divine Wisdom

"Divine Wisdom is about the process of renewal, expansion, and becoming consciously aware and awakened." –BT

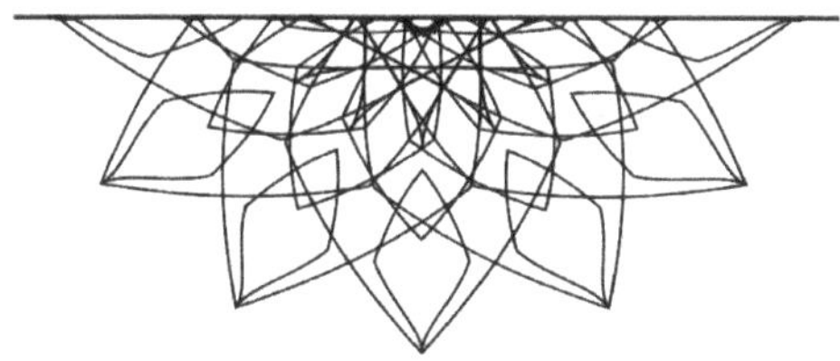

"I am the Light of Divine Wisdom. Through this Sacred Truth, I remember I have an all-knowing, internal guidance, and sacred awareness at all times."

How to Develop Divine Wisdom

Divine Wisdom is where we transcend the duality of looking at ourselves as human beings or Spiritual beings. The truth is there is no separation between the two. We are not separate from Spirit, nor are we separate from each other.

REMEMBER WHO YOU ARE

- Do you see yourself as a Divine being and welcome the influence of Spirit in all that you do?
- Do you recognize that there is no difference between the Light that surrounds you and the Light that you are?
- What are some experiences you have had that you know were Divinely guided/co-created with Spirit? Describe them.

CO-CREATE YOUR LIFE

- Where in your life are you floundering?
- Can you pause and observe the situation? Scope out and witness your actions.
- Are you loving into the experience?
- Are you asking for Divine assistance and co-creating? Remember, it is a giving and receiving.
- Resist the impulse to always "do something" and trust that with reflection, stillness, and silence, a solution will come forward.

BE THE OBSERVER OF YOUR DREAMS

- Most intuitive downloads happen while you sleep because your ego and your analytical brain are on pause. This allows the truth to come through.
- Dreams tell a story of how you authentically feel. Once again, we need to pull back and decode their messages.
- WRITE YOUR DREAMS DOWN IMMEDIATELY! Very important details get lost if you wait.
- Review what you wrote down several times and highlight what stands out to you. These details have meaning and symbolism.

SOUL WRITING

- I always begin by asking Spirit, "What do I need to know today or about this particular situation?"
- Listening takes practice and patience. Just begin to write down anything and everything you are feeling.
- How do you decipher between the ego and true Divine Wisdom? Remember, Divine Wisdom is expansive. Egoic thoughts are filled with structure, limitations, and fear.

THERE'S MAGIC IN THE PAUSE

- Get comfortable with being in silence. It is the only way to hear your Divine Inner Wisdom. Turn off the TV, music, and podcasts. Separate yourself from social media.
- The only way to hear your Divinity speaking is to practice times of pause and silence. This could be in seated meditation, forest walking, knitting, digging in the garden, or even doing the dishes.
- Finding your moment of Zen is all about being able to still the mind, breathe deeply, calm the body, and listen to its wisdom.
- What is your Divine Inner Wisdom trying to communicate?

HIT UNSUBSCRIBE

- Quit accepting and agreeing to all the limiting beliefs you have been carrying around with you.
- Clear the clutter in your inbox/brain/ego.
- Notice how your thoughts and beliefs have made you feel throughout your life.
- Find that place of expanded awareness, meaning pulling back all layers and being completely honest with yourself.
- Observe your experiences without judgment or attachment.
- When you finally allow the voice of Spirit to communicate, IT IS LIBERATING.
- What limiting beliefs are you able to recognize and release?

ADDITIONAL THOUGHTS & FEELINGS

ADDITIONAL THOUGHTS & FEELINGS

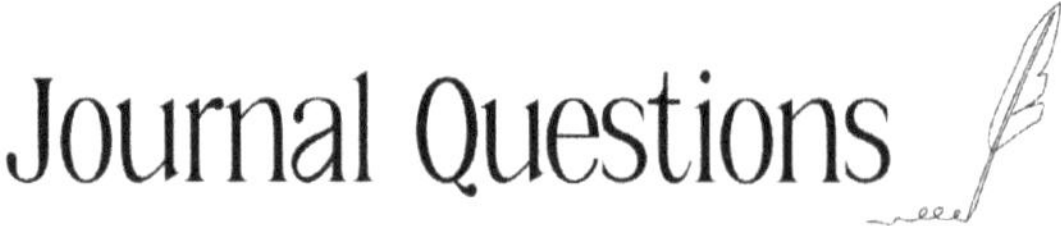

Journal Questions

DO YOU FIND YOU ARE INDECISIVE?

- If so, what is the root of your indecision?
- Can you tap into your inner wisdom to help you find clarity?

DO YOU FEEL STUCK WITH NO VISION FOR YOURSELF?

- Write down your fears about moving forward.
- Then, write down how expansive it feels when you allow yourself to daydream about moving forward.

DO YOU FEEL LOST ON YOUR SPIRITUAL PATH OR LIFE PURPOSE?

Take a minute to daydream and write down what truly inspires you. You may need to dig back into your childhood.

DO YOU FEEL YOU ARE LIVING PARTIALLY OR ENTIRELY IN A FANTASY OR DAYDREAM STATE AND ARE UNCOMFORTABLE LIVING AND BEING PRESENT IN YOUR DAILY LIFE?

- What makes you uncomfortable?
- What in your life are you avoiding?

DO YOU FEEL OPEN TO A HIGHER POWER?

- Everyone has a different view of what a "higher power" looks like, so keep your heart open to what that is for you.
- Take a minute to write about what you love, and you may just find your higher power there. (For example, I connect with my higher power the best when I am in water. I feel the resonance of Spirit in water.)
- How does it come in for you?
- Write about how it feels.

DO YOU RECOGNIZE YOUR ABILITY TO CO-CREATE WITH YOUR DIVINE WISDOM?

- Can you feel the emotional difference between your intuition and intellect?
- Does your intuition reveal a more profound level of truth?

WHAT BELIEFS AND ATTITUDES IN YOURSELF WOULD YOU LIKE TO CHANGE?

- Can you commit to making those changes?
- Do you procrastinate taking action even though you recognize this change would benefit your life?
- Can you identify your reasons or fears for not taking action?

ADDITIONAL THOUGHTS & FEELINGS

ADDITIONAL THOUGHTS & FEELINGS

ADDITIONAL THOUGHTS & FEELINGS

Divine Light

"I used to seek the Light.
I decided to become the Light instead." –BT

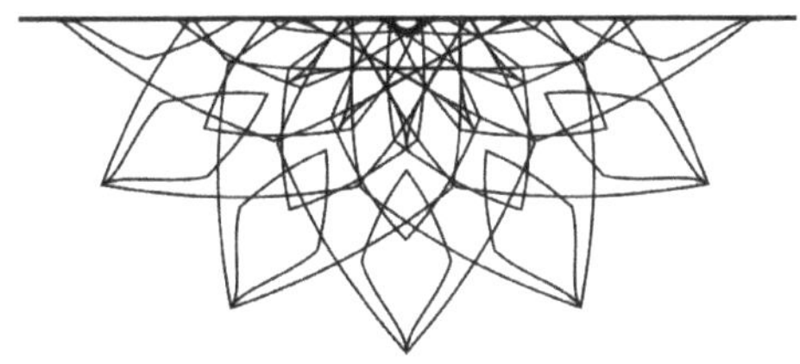

"I am Divine Light. Through this Sacred Truth, I am expanding my Light body and knowing my connection to all things."

How to Live in Divine Light

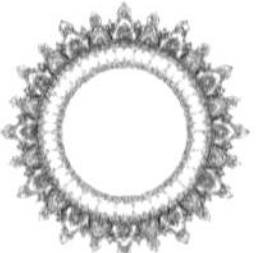

The crown chakra is the gateway to Divine Consciousness. The Sacred Divine Intention for your crown chakra is to hold yourself in a God state at all times. This Divine Truth reminds us that we are not separate from each other, as we learned in the previous chapter. Living in a God state and integrating this Sacred Truth means knowing we are also not separate from Spirit. Rather, we are one with Spirit. Spirit is not only within us but *is* us. We are one with each other, the Universe, and Spirit––and we are love.

STAND IN YOUR TRUTH

- Standing in truth is knowing that it is impossible to be separate from Spirit and each other.
- Living in presence and in the Light calls for constant attunement.
- The gift of presence is that our hearts KNOW this unbreakable connection to each other and to Spirit.
- What does it feel like when you are living in presence?
- What are ways for you to stay attuned?

The Seven Stages of Presence

In the following exercise, I am taking all of the Divine Affirmations and integrating them with the breath for more powerful healing. It's important to speak these affirmations out loud. Remember that words carry a vibration, and hearing these affirmations helps the truth harmonize and ground within your body. **THESE EXERCISES ARE RECORDED. https://bit.ly/463gmxS. QR Code at the bottom of this page.**

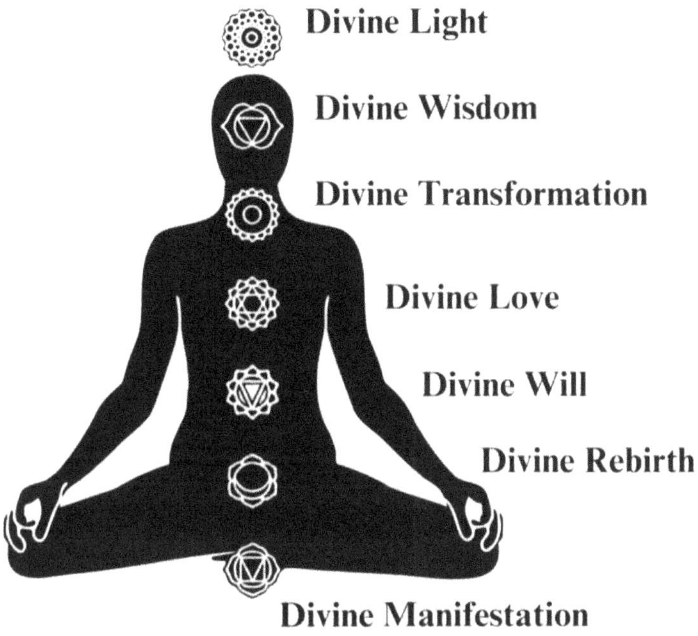

Divine Light

Divine Wisdom

Divine Transformation

Divine Love

Divine Will

Divine Rebirth

Divine Manifestation

LET'S BEGIN WITH A BASIC GROUNDING BREATH EXERCISE

Visualize with each breath are millions of rainbow ray Spirit particles lighting up every cell in our body.

- Sit comfortably with your eyes closed. Breathe deeply and steadily throughout this exercise. Keep the spine straight & feet or sitting bones grounded to the floor.
- Begin by visualizing and inhaling a stream of energy or a cord running down from the base of the spine. Feel it move down through the floor and into the earth. Visualize it running down and spreading out like the roots of a tree, anchoring and grounding deeper and deeper through all of the layers of the earth until you have finally reached the crystalline core of the earth.
- Allow the cord to anchor into the center of the earth.
- Give a greeting and gratitude to Mama Gaia.
- Now, bring your awareness to a higher level of the earth and begin to allow the stability of the earth's energy to rise with your next inhale back up the roots you set. Using your breath, draw that energy back up and into your feet, up your legs, and into the base of your spine/1st chakra/Muladhara.
- Feel the earth's energy stream up from the earth and into your body. Just allow it to mix there with your body's life force. Allow your body to distribute this energy where it needs to go.
- Enjoy the stability you feel. (This constitutes the grounding aspect of this exercise. Grounding can be done anytime and should be done frequently.)
- After bringing earth energy in to support and harmonize with the body, move your attention to the crown chakra/7th chakra (located at the top of your head). With your attention and focus, allow this energy center to open and expand.
- Honoring Divine Spirit, visualize a beautiful, expansive orb of white light just above your head.
- With your breath, begin to draw that light into the crown chakra. From the crown chakra, bring the light into your 6th chakra (the space between your eyebrows). Then pull the light into your 5th chakra/throat chakra. Finally, pull the light from your throat to your 4th chakra/heart center.
- Hold the light in that space and feel it expand with each breath. As it gets larger, it clears and opens space, releasing stress, anxiety, and all unwanted emotions and filling your physical body with light, peace, and a pure sense of calm.

SEVEN STAGES OF PRESENCE EXERCISE
ONCE WE KNOW AND HOLD THE SEVEN SACRED TRUTHS WITHIN OUR HEARTS, WE ARE PREPARED TO AWAKEN TO THE *I AM.*

By breathing the Light from our oversoul (the magnificent orb of Light that sits about 18 inches above your head and holds the blueprint to your perfection) into the crown chakra (at the top of the head), then guiding it into the chakra pillar (located along the spine), and grounding this sacred Light into the earth, we create a continuum of all our conscious Sacred Intentions.

- Sitting up or lying down with your spine straight, gently breathe into your crown chakra with a long, slow, steady breath through the nose. Pause and hold the breath in your body once your lungs are full. Slowly exhale through your nose. Then say, "I am Divine Light." It's important to say this out loud so the vibration of your words is not only heard but deeply felt. Repeat these steps three times to allow better integration of the Light. Finally, breathe from your crown chakra at the top of your head down to the first chakra at the tip of your tailbone. Again, breathe slowly through the nose. Pause and hold your breath. Gently exhale. In doing this, you are expanding your Light Body and feeling the connection to all things.

- Following the same method as above, breathe into the sixth chakra (third eye), which is the space between your eyebrows along your brow bone. Pause and hold the breath. On the exhale, say, "I am the Light of Divine Loving Wisdom." This helps you remember that you have a higher, all-knowing, all-wise, all-seeing awareness at all times. Please repeat this three times.

- Breathe into your fifth chakra, located at the base of your neck. Pause and hold the breath. On the exhale, say, "I am the Light of Divine Transformation and self-expression." This reminds you that with every breath, you have the ability to transform because within each breath is the Light of Spirit. Every word you speak holds the resonance of love and compassion. Please repeat this three times.

- Breathe into your fourth chakra, in the center of your heart. Pause and hold the breath. On the exhale, say, "I am the Light of Divine Love." Remember that the Light and love within your heart supersedes all fear and heals through unconditional love. Please repeat this three times.

- Breathe into your third chakra, located in the solar plexus/diaphragm. Pause and hold the breath. On the exhale, say, "I am the Light of Divine Will." The Light of Divine Will within me allows me to supersede my ego and surrender to the truth, thus allowing me to feel the beauty, bliss, and perfection in all things. Please repeat this three times.

- Breathe into your second chakra, located just below the navel. Pause and hold the breath. On the exhale, say, "I am the Light of Divine Rebirth." Through this truth, I have all potential to transform, regenerate, renew, and reawaken all things. Please repeat this three times.
- Breathe into your first chakra, located at the base of the spine. On the exhale, say, "I am the Light of Divine Manifestation." Through these truths, I have created a sacred vessel to hold this Light. It is completely grounded and integrated within both my Light body and physical body. All is love and requires nothing else. "And so it is, and so it shall be." Please repeat this three times.

ADDITIONAL THOUGHTS & FEELINGS FROM THESE EXERCISES

ADDITIONAL THOUGHTS & FEELINGS

Journal Questions

DO YOU FEEL A CONNECTION TO A HIGHER POWER?

If not, what is the barrier preventing you from allowing this relationship?

DO YOU FEEL LIKE YOU HAVE A DIVINE PURPOSE IN THIS LIFETIME?

- What does your gift to the world look like?
- This does not need to be a grand gesture. Being an example of human kindness or a guardian of the earth fulfills an extraordinary purpose.

HOW CAN YOU DO MORE OF WHAT INSPIRES YOU TO CONTINUALLY SEEK AND LIVE IN YOUR PURPOSE?

Are there ways you can simplify your life so you live less in the distractions of the material world and more in your Divinity?

HOW CAN YOU BE OF SERVICE TO OTHERS?

Once again, this does not have to be a grand gesture. Simply opening the door and offering a kind welcome can be a day changer for someone else.

WHEN AND HOW CAN YOU INCORPORATE DAILY SILENCE, PRAYER, OR MEDITATION TIME?

What allows you to go internal? Sometimes we need to occupy our body with movement in order to calm the mind and allow the heart to sing (i.e., forest walking, running, swimming, dancing, yoga).

DO YOU HAVE SPIRITUAL TRUTHS THAT YOU LIVE BY?

We identify these truths because they are based in love.

DO YOU SEEK DIVINE GUIDANCE DURING MEDITATION?

- Try asking, "What do I need to know?" Then, pause and receive the answer.
- Are you open that this response may not be precisely what you asked for but may actually turn out to be better?
- Consider ending your time of silence and meditation (prayer) time with gratitude, then journal about it.

ARE YOU DEVOTED TO A PARTICULAR SPIRITUAL PATH? IF NOT, DO YOU FEEL THE NEED TO FIND ONE?

Do you fear expanding your Spiritual path and creating a closer relationship with the Divine because of changes it might trigger in your life?

DO YOU SPEND TOO MUCH TIME IN MEDITATION AND IN THE SPIRIT WORLD, AVOIDING OR NOT TENDING TO YOUR DAILY PHYSICAL NEEDS?

- Can you identify what is making you uncomfortable in your physical existence?
- What would bring more balance into your life?

ADDITIONAL THOUGHTS & FEELINGS

ADDITIONAL THOUGHTS & FEELINGS

ADDITIONAL THOUGHTS & FEELINGS

ADDITIONAL THOUGHTS & FEELINGS

ADDITIONAL THOUGHTS & FEELINGS

Let's Manifest!

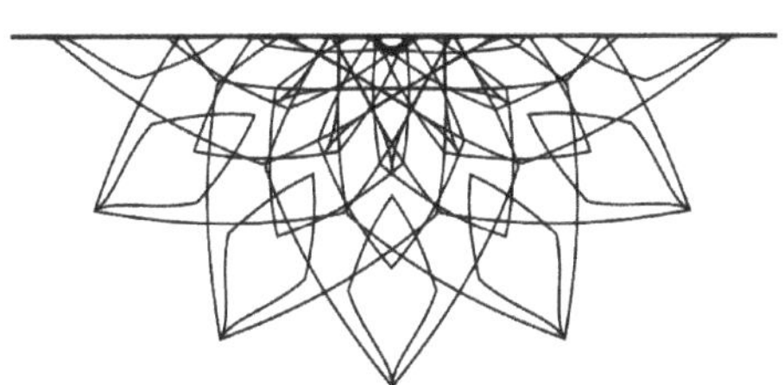

THINK BACK THROUGHOUT YOUR LIFE. WHAT IS SOMETHING THAT YOU ALWAYS WANTED AND YOU WERE ACTUALLY ABLE TO MANIFEST?

- How did it feel to bring this gift forward?
- How did you release limiting beliefs and know you could do it?

ALL MANIFESTATIONS MUST COME FROM THE HEART

- What is something that your heart truly desires?
- Write or pray about it.
- Ask Spirit for guidance.
- Trust that your intention has been heard and answered.
- Stay in a place of pause and silence in order to receive.
- Get out of the way and allow Spirit to present you with the perfect manifestation of your desire.
- Journal about the journey.

MANIFESTING MIRACLES REQUIRES US TO SYNCHRONIZE WITH THE LIFE FORCE OF THE DIVINE AND OUR LOVED ONES ON THE OTHER SIDE

- Remember, synchronicities occur when your vibration matches that of something else.
- Each day, write down any synchronicities you notice.

ADDITIONAL THOUGHTS & FEELINGS

ADDITIONAL THOUGHTS & FEELINGS

ADDITIONAL THOUGHTS & FEELINGS

In Light and Love!

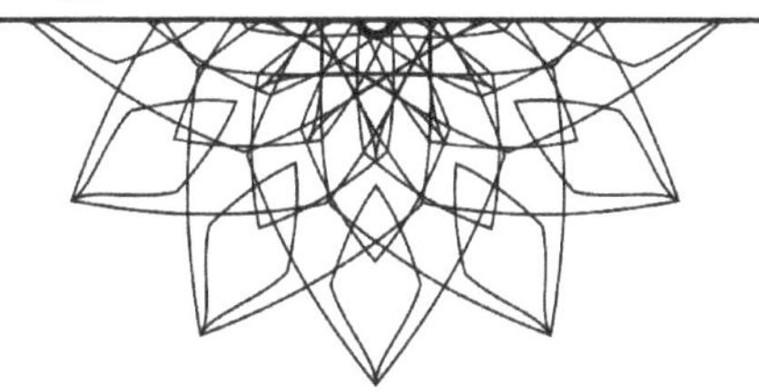

I sincerely hope you found this workbook helpful because, as I said in *Stand in Your Truth,*

"We are here to be ministering angels for each other, so go forth to love and to serve for the highest and best good of all.

Collectively, as one person rises, we all rise."

Please know that I am sending you so much love. If you need any support, I'd love to work with you in either an in-person or virtual healing session.

Suzy Schaaf

SCHEDULE A HEALING SESSION
https://bit.ly/3YzNI2K

www.ingramcontent.com/pod-product-compliance
Lightning Source LLC
Chambersburg PA
CBHW040731120726
48010CB00002B/80

* 9 7 9 8 2 1 8 4 1 7 5 1 2 *